The TLC Diet Transformation

Lose Weight, Lower Cholesterol and Transform Your Life With the TLC Diet (Before It Is Too Late)!

RON KNESS

ISBN-13: 978-1544161389

ISBN-10: 1544161387

Contents

Disclaimer

This publication is for informational purposes only and is not intended as medical advice. Medical advice should always be obtained from a qualified medical professional for any health conditions or symptoms associated with them.

Every possible effort has been made in preparing and researching this material. We make no warranties with respect to the accuracy, applicability of its contents or any omissions.

See your healthcare professional before starting any diet, health or exercise program!

Introduction

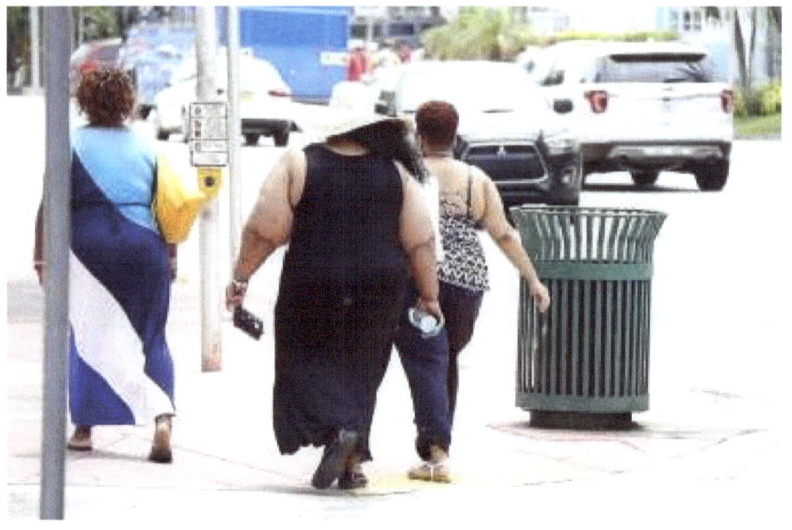

Let's start this beginners' guide on the TLC diet with a little mental exercise. When you go out, look around you and tell me what you see. I bet you will see an abundance of fast food restaurants and guess what's in front of them? You guessed it … a never-ending line of people.

Fast food joints are known for serving up a dish of unhealthy food – unhealthy food that people continue to consume. Why? Three reasons: 1)Because they can! 2) Because they don't know better. 3) Because they don't care.

People choose fast food because they live a busy life and are under the impression that they can't go home and cook a healthy meal, because it will take hours to do.

This unhealthy lifestyle leads to obesity.

The health risks of being obese include:

- Heart disease

- Type 2 diabetes

- Osteoarthritis

- Nonalcoholic fatty liver disease

- High blood pressure

- Stroke

Reasons People Are Unhealthy

- Most work available is white-collar and think they don't have time to cook

- Children now spend more time playing digital games instead of playing outside thus burning fewer calories

- The foods low-income families think they can afford are unhealthy; actually the opposite is true

- The serving sizes of unhealthy drinks and fast food have increased

- People buy more fast food and prepare fewer meals in their kitchen due to a lack of knowledge about food and its preparation

This list could go on and on …

There's an old Chinese proverb that does a good job at explaining why we need to watch what we put in our mouths. "When you're thirsty, it's too late to dig a well."

What this is saying is that you should not wait until you have an illness to start eating healthy, because by then, it may be too late.

The Need For Health In The Modern Age

There are many important reasons why you should get in shape today. What "getting in shape" means to me is you have strength, a baseline cardiovascular capacity, muscular endurance and flexibility, which all leads to a healthier life.

Believe it or not, the 21st century conditions could be damaging your health and you don't even realize it. Let's have a look at some of these modern-day health conditions being experienced ...

Toasted Skin Syndrome

Have you ever heard of this? Have you ever balanced your laptop on your knees for a long period of time? Believe it or not, it can leave you with discolored skin!

The heat generated by your laptop, can cause a rash that is similar to someone that has huddled to close to a heater in order to stay warm. Mind you, this has nothing to do with dieting or exercise – this is just showing you how our health is being affected in the modern age by technology.

Time Poverty

Oh yes, good old time poverty – so many of us are a victim of this. With family, work, running a home, and trying to take care of everything, we hardly find time to sit down and pause for a nice breath of fresh air. The more we rush, the further we struggle to meet deadlines we have imposed. The result? Our health. We deal with everything from insomnia, stress, depression and poor diet, which leads to obesity and many other health related issues. Many of us are simply doing too much and in return, this is taking a major toll on our health and well-being.

Living in Fear

Many will refer to this as "the 21st century fear." Here we are, constantly staring at the threat of floods, disease, crime, hurricanes, terrorist attacks, toxic chemicals in food and so much more. We're constantly focusing on those fears. We have become so worried about the things that "might" happen to the point that we have stopped enjoying life that is taking place in front of us. As you may already know, too much worry isn't good for your health.

We may not be able to help you with toasted skin syndrome, other than tell you not to place your laptop on your lap for a prolonged time, but we may be able to help you with time poverty. This is where the TLC diet is going to come into play.

You see, in the modern day scenario, everything comes at a price. Our days and nights are filled with hectic schedules, unavoidable deadlines and innumerable hours of stress and excessive workload. With so much already on our plate, we cease to care about the food what we consume at the end of a long tiring day.

Most often, we are too tired to cook a healthy, nutritious meal post work and end up opting for the easier option: fast food and processed items. With the technology available today, everything is just a click of a mouse or a phone call away.

As we previously stated, most people settle for a comforting double cheese burger, pizza or fries to hush their roaring stomach every day. Although these food choices offer oodles of contentment and comfort, eventually they bring forth drastic side effects. Overtime, with continuous consumption, unhealthy food choices lead to several modern day ailments, such as diabetes, obesity, hypertension, depression, anxiety, high cholesterol and other health related concerns.

Most of these complaints start out small but gradually turn into unavoidable chronic conditions. The best deterrent is to wake up now, take action and prevent such ailments from deteriorating your health and fitness in the first place. Whatever diet changes you make today will help improve your health. Even if you are already afflicted with one or more of the above conditions. But you have to start now!

For all those facing similar conditions, this short beginner's guide brings a suitable solution to combat the most frequent of our modern day health problems. It introduces the concept of the TLC Diet or the Therapeutic Lifestyle Changes program.

Are you ready? Let's get started...

What Exactly Is The TLC Diet?

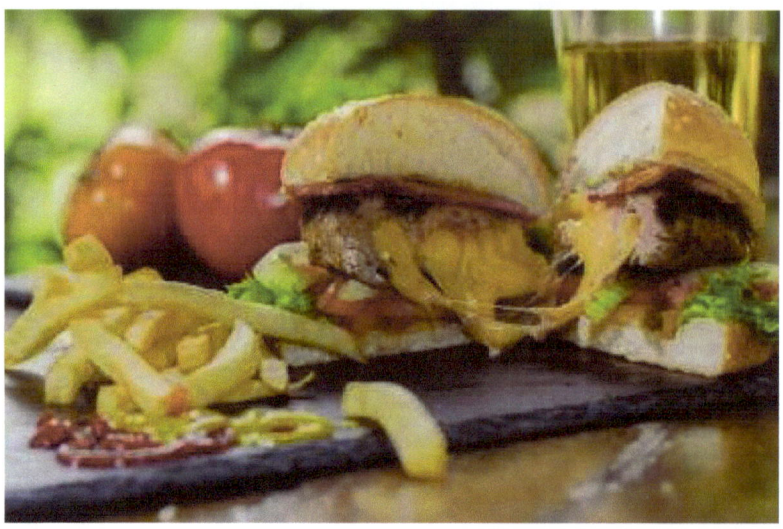

This healthy eating diet focuses mainly on modifying the increasing or already hyped levels of cholesterol.

When the body contains an excessive level of cholesterol, over time it weakens the heart and causes several fatal conditions, like a sudden heart attack and stroke among other serious cardiovascular conditions.

It is highly recommended to take charge of your body and health before it worsens to a point where it is beyond repair.

This diet encourages healthy measures to lower cholesterol levels by means of diet, exercise and other related methods. It also brings successful weight loss in its wake. For all those struggling with weight loss or health conditions, the TLC diet is a great way to kick start your way to good health and wellbeing.

The Therapeutic Lifestyle Changes diet was initially coined by the NATIONAL Heart, Lung and Blood Institute in the year 2001. Due to its beneficial nature, the diet has also been approved and encouraged by the American Heart Association.

The diet aims at reducing the LDL levels of cholesterol, also known as the bad cholesterol, which is held responsible for triggering cardio vascular complications.

The diet focuses mainly on healthy food options that have been coupled with suitable exercise and required lifestyle changes to help speed the process of recovery without any medications.

It not just keeps the LDL levels in control, but also works towards providing the body the right level of HDL or the good healthy cholesterol that is required by the body for proper functioning, induced growth and development.

Although the diet does bring about some weight loss in its process, the goal is improved health by controlling cholesterol more than focusing solely on losing weight.

Well that's a quick overview of what the TLC diet is, over the next few chapters we will cover exactly what cholesterol is, the benefits of starting a TLC diet program and what foods you need to include in your everyday diet.

All About Cholesterol

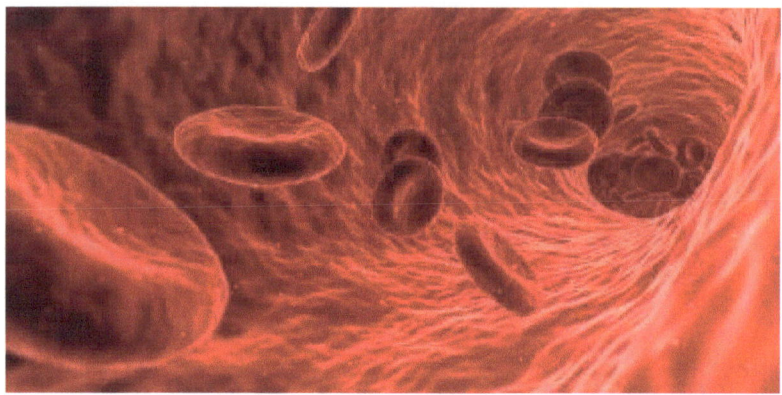

Again, and again, food and our diet has been named as the major culprit for causing health problems around the world.

High blood pressure or hypertension is now a very big problem. It is considered the number one killer in America, and perhaps in many other countries around the world.

Undoubtedly, a person with a high blood pressure is facing many risks in relation to health. There are many complications and diseases associated with having high blood pressure.   The truth of the matter is this trend is quite unsurprising. With the fashion in which we are eating nowadays, it is easy to see why high blood pressure is a problem. Processed and fast food is normally high in sodium which is a major contributor to hypertension.

Considering the current eating trends around the world, it is inevitable that health has suffered. We all eat too much of the wrong things. The fast-food culture is proving to be surprisingly strong. Many of us prefer to eat junk food because it is convenient and easily available.

Children are growing obese and adults are growing unhealthy because of it. Our current culture makes it difficult for us to make healthy choices. The current lifestyle choices of modern man are often very unhealthy.

Furthermore, it gets even more confusing for people nowadays because there are so many fly-by-night diet trends and diet rules. It gets difficult to figure out which diets are truly beneficial to your health and which ones are just a passing fad.

There are an abundance of different kinds of diets to choose from, it gets difficult to pick which one will be right for you.

And it seems as though some people are more concerned about their appearance, but are not truly concerned about their health. In effect, you have teenagers who choose to starve themselves in order to look like the people they see in magazines. Health is more than just about having a nice body. It means having a body which functions properly. And you can have both; it is not that hard to do, but may take more time.

As said earlier, high blood pressure is a serious problem. It prevents your body from functioning properly, and it might also lead to the development of other diseases. The number of people who are suffering from high blood pressure is growing by the day and it's surprising that we aren't taking this problem as seriously as we should. Many are already suffering and many more will suffer if the proper steps are not taken.

If you know that you have high blood pressure, don't ignore it! It can lead to serious complications which could possibly damage your health and your body permanently. If you don't get the proper medical attention that you need, you might end up with very serious problems or even die as a result of it.

The good news is that there is no reason for you to panic. You can easily take control of the situation if you can make a commitment to a healthier lifestyle.

Why Does Cholesterol Matter?

For the past few decades or so, cholesterol was always seen as the enemy. It was seen as the reason for heart failures and it was blamed for many things. People feared cholesterol, and the rule in every household was to keep it as low as possible.

While there are certain studies which now claim that cholesterol should not be demonized, it should still be monitored well to ensure that a person's body will continue to function well.

Here's a little surprise, you actually need cholesterol in your body. It is essential to life and is needed by cell membranes.

It is classified as a lipid and it is found in most animals. Even though it is a fat, it is essential to certain metabolic processes. In fact, most of our cholesterol is produced by the liver and most of the cells in our bodies. It helps in many biological processes like the absorption of vitamin D.

Cholesterol is useful but it has to be controlled. Health experts recommend that triglyceride levels (which in part measure both the good and bad cholesterol among other things) should not exceed 150 milligrams per deciliter. Those with pre-existing risk factors should aim for number lower than 150. Unfortunately for many, it is just a number - a number that many of us choose to ignore. And as a result, many have a high cholesterol count because of it.

If a person has too much cholesterol circulating in his or her bloodstream, it can get quite dangerous. Too much cholesterol can cause blood vessels to narrow, and eventually, be blocked. When blood vessels are blocked, it can lead to many different diseases like stroke or various heart diseases – some of which can be fatal.

There are many factors which affect a person's cholesterol levels. Some people are more likely to have high-blood pressure because of genetics and family background. Others may have it because of a related medical condition like an under active thyroid gland, overconsumption of alcohol and obesity. Some risk factors are more dangerous than others and should be taken in to account.

It is important to look at a person's overall lifestyle in order to figure out the best possible solution to the problem.

Perhaps the most noticeable and controllable factor in preventing high blood pressure is monitoring a person's diet. While people's bodies might react differently even if they eat the same thing, switching to more health-conscious food choices will very likely improve a person's health conditions.

At the very least, it will not hurt to switch to a healthier eating plan! Generally speaking, those who eat foods that are low in saturated fat can really help improve their health overall.

The majority of those who have high blood pressure do not show the symptoms of the condition ... yet. People over twenty years of age should ideally have their blood pressure checked at least once every year during their annual physical if they are in the high risk group. Those with good numbers may be able to get tested less frequently, but should still do it to ensure that they stay in good condition. Consult your doctor or health care provider to find out how often you should take the test.

Major Benefits of the TLC Diet

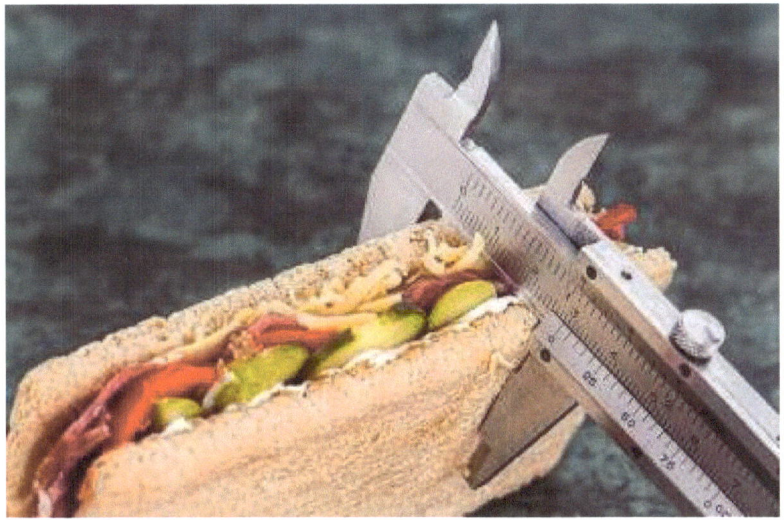

Are you starting to think the TLC diet is for you? Well if so then take a look at the major benefits if you decide to follow this way of eating ...

1. Easy to Follow

This healthy diet is simple and easy to follow   There are no special kinds of foods that you need to cook. There is no need to learn a new recipe. You don't need to buy special and expensive ingredients. The diet is simple, straightforward and inexpensive.   The meals are easy to prepare. Since you don't need to strictly follow a specific meal plan, you have the freedom to modify the recipes per what is available for you.

Since this diet will allow you to modify your meals, it is also possible to adjust it if you are vegetarian or if you want it to be gluten-free. The important thing is to learn how to eat generally within the guidelines of the diet. Once you know and understand the basic principles which make the diet so effective, it will undoubtedly be much easier for you to modify the diet in accordance with your individual needs.

2. It is Proven Effective

The diet is healthy and proven effective   The effects of the TLC diet are long-term. This is because rather than providing a quick-fix solution to the problem, the TLC diet encourages positive changes in a person's lifestyle – changes you can live with for the rest of your life. The true secret of maintaining a healthy lifestyle is knowing how to keep eating healthy and how to continue exercising for a long time. Rather than a race, think of health as a marathon. It cannot be rushed and it must be taken slowly but surely.

The reason other diets fail is because they are so extreme and restrictive, people can't stay on them for very long. So they keep going from one diet to another trying to find one that works for them. The TLC Diet is the holy grail when compared to the rest of the diets out there. Later in the book you can read a comparison between the TLC Diet and a few of the more popular ones.

3. Educates People

The TLC diet actually educates people.   With the TLC diet, a person is made aware of what he or she should eat and drink.

A person learns how to choose what is healthy. This means knowing how to shop for healthy items, how to read labels and how to prepare meals in a healthy way. A person will also know how to compute how much saturated fat is recommended verses how much is actually consumed. And how to calculate how much trans fats are in a product when the nutrition label says it has none. We've included a separate chapter on how to read a nutrition label and know what you are reading.

Unlike some other diets, you will not be told what you should eat in every single meal. Therefore, it is up to a person to choose his or her meals according to what he or she learns.

Well those are just a few of the main benefits gained by following the principles of the TLC Diet.

In the next part we will look more specifically at what to eat and how to get your proper nutrients in.

Nutrition and What To Eat On the TLC Diet

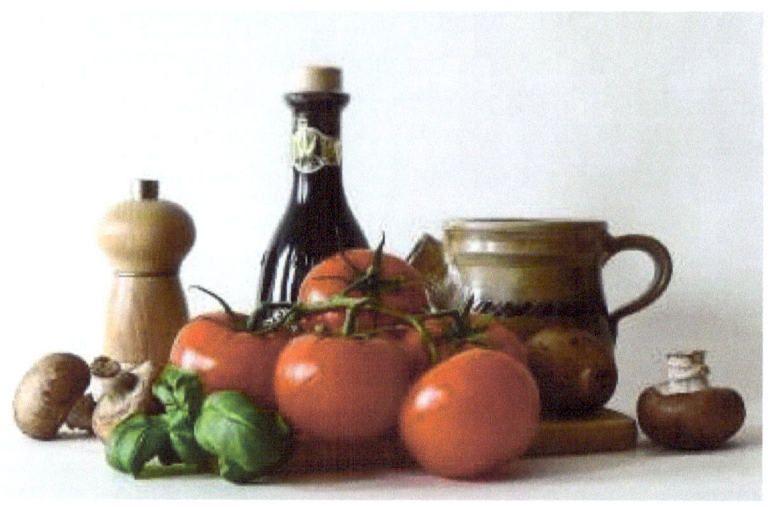

To lower your cholesterol levels, there's no getting around the fact that you must know something about the nutritional value of the food you put in your mouth.

The TLC program's major focus is to create a nutritious way of eating that will provide the correct nutrients and will reduce the amount of saturated fat you eat.

These saturated fats are the ones that elevate your cholesterol levels. First you want to reduce the foods high in saturated fats, like fatty cuts of meat and whole milk products you eat.

You will also have to replace some of the animal fats and choose some healthy, monounsaturated oils – olive oil, for example.

Another good option is choosing a fatty acid supplement like Omega-3. These fats will keep the good cholesterol up and lower the bad one.

The types of food you eat can be as important as their calorie content. What is good for one person may not be the same for the other. It is thus important to understand your metabolic system and nutritional needs.

What are calories?

There is so much hype surrounding calories these days. All of us know that in order to lose weight, we must burn more calories than we eat. But what exactly are calories? In simple words, calories are units of energy in food or drinks required by the body to perform its functions. The amount of calories needed by your body depends in part on the amount of energy required by your body to keep warm and alive – known as your Basal Metabolic Rate or BMR.

This is exactly what your body needs, irrespective of your activities or other factors dictating the number of calories you burn each day. Typically, the larger an individual, the greater their caloric need is or their BMR.

If your body needs, for example, 2,000 calories today, it will require the same amount tomorrow and the next day and so on. However, the BMR does vary from person to person, depending on the body size, age and amount of work you do ... just to name a few of the factors affecting the number of calories burned.

What Can You Eat?

The TLC program is based on consuming a wide array of different foods but in doing so, getting a proper ratio of nutrients to fuel your body effectively. Food choices are not restricted per se, but must be consumed in a limited amount. These amounts are sometimes a percentage of your total calorie intake for each day.

- Saturated fat - Less than 7 % of total calories

- Polyunsaturated fat - Up to 10 % of total calories

- Monounsaturated fat - Up to 20 % of total calories

- Carbohydrate - 50 % to 60 % of total calories

- Soluble fiber - At least 5 to 10 grams a day

- Protein Approximately - 15 % of total calories

Fat

The biggest part of TLC diet program is about fats and is where we are going to focus our attention on in this beginner's guide. If you get the correct amount of good fats in your diet, most of the other things will fall into place (carbs, protein & fiber).

These fats can help you fight those cholesterol levels, or help you feed them. You have to learn what fat actually is in order to defeat it – get to know your enemy before fighting it!

Fat seems to be a dreaded word for most of us. But have you ever wondered why there is so much hue and cry about fat? First, I need you to understand this.

Dietary fat is different than your body fat.

It appears that the lack of knowledge of nutrition scares most people into thinking dietary fat is bad. It can be considered a word and image association where you hear the word "fat" and automatically associate it with the fat on your belly. Automatically you think, "Uh oh, I don't want any more fat on my stomach, I don't want that food if it has fat." So, is a low-fat diet a solution for all ills?

Well, before answering this question, it is important to find whether you are eating healthy fats or not. Healthy fats include seeds, nuts, and unrefined oils, along with naturally occurring fats in vegetables and meats. As with most things food connected, the key lies in maintaining moderation and optimizing nutritional benefits. Experts recommend that fats and oil should suffice for at least 10–40 percent of your regular energy needs.

Though fats have earned a poor reputation for their effect on heart health and obesity, some fat is ESSENTIAL for health and wellbeing.

Fats help in the absorption of carotenoids and fat-soluble vitamins - A, D, E, K. Without a proper amount of fat to metabolize these vitamins, they go through your body unused and you derive no useful nutritional benefit from them. Essential fatty acids needed by the body, which it cannot make on its own, such as omega-3, is an unsaturated fat that we must consume from our diets mainly found in fish.

Fats have the potential to harm as well as help our health; depending on their fatty acid composition, their nutritional value, and their condition.

When used in a natural, unadulterated state, fat offers optimal nutritional benefits. On the other hand, a very-low-fat diet can compromise our health and ability to lose weight.

Fatty Acids

When you eat food, the fat comprised in the food is known as fatty acids. Typically considered "good fats," fatty acids are known as the building blocks of many cellular structures and hormonal patterns in the human body.

Healthy Nuts, Seeds, Fats And Oils

Foods high in healthy unsaturated fatty acids include these nuts, seeds and oils:

- Almonds

- Pistachios

- Walnuts

- Hazelnuts

- Sesame Seeds

- Pecans

- Brazil Nuts

- Sunflower Seeds

- Macadamia Nuts

- Cashews

- Peanuts

- Pumpkin Seeds

- Chia Seeds

Fats and oils to use:

- Almond Oil

- Red Palm Oil

- Extra Virgin Olive Oil

- Grape seed oil

- Sesame Oil

- Flax Seed Oil

- Macadamia Nut Oil

- Hemp

- Coconut Oil

- Safflower Oil

These fatty acids help in the transfer of oxygen to different parts of the body through the bloodstream. These fats help keep skin healthy, thus preventing signs of early aging. They also promote cell membrane development and are essential for strong organs and tissue.

They help the body process cholesterol and rid the arteries of plaque or cholesterol build-up. Fatty acids boost the functioning of adrenal and thyroid glands, thus helping regulate weight.

Without them in the proper quantity, your body cannot function at its optimal level.

How to Read a Food Nutrition Label

Nutrition Facts

Serving Size 8 oz (227 g/8 oz)
Servings Per Container About 3

Amount Per Serving

Calories 180   Calories from Fat 60

	% Daily Value*
Total Fat 6g	10 %
Saturated Fat 1g	5 %
Trans Fat 0g	
Cholesterol 5mg	2 %
Sodium 75mg	3 %
Total Carbohydrate 26g	9 %
Dietary Fiber 5g	19 %
Sugars 11g	
Protein 8g	

One of the most important things you can do for your own nutrition is to know what you're eating. In recent years, food labels have become much more user friendly and you really can know exactly what you're putting in your body.

Your relationship with food is very important. What you eat can help to give you energy, improve your immunity, and allow you to combat many diseases. But it can also do the opposite – leave you feeling weak and even cause disease.

But if you've never given your food much thought, reading food labels can be intimidating. There's a lot of information there. Deciding which information is important and which isn't can be challenging. Once you know the basics, though, you'll read those labels with confidence.

Be Smart about Serving Size

Begin with looking at the serving size on the label. Sometimes people miss this part and then have an inaccurate idea of what's actually in the food. For example, if you have a can of soup and the label says it's 2 servings, that means that the information on the label would be doubled if you ate the whole can.

Labels have gotten better in the recent past. For example, a can of soda used to be 1.5 or 2 servings. But now when you look at the label, one can of soda is a whole serving because most people will drink the entire thing. A 20 oz. bottle, though, is more than 2 servings.

Calorie Breakdown

Once you know the serving size, you're ready to move on to looking at the quality of the food you're eating. The most obvious information you can get from your food label is about the breakdown of calories.

The label will tell you how many calories are in each serving. Calories are the measurement of energy. Depending on the type of calories, dictates how long it will take to break down the item. If most of the calories come from a simple carb like sugar, the breakdown will be fast. If from complex carbs, such as whole grain, it will be slow. Comple3x carbs keep you feeling fuller longer thus reducing your urge to eat as soon.

Your metabolism is the measure of how much energy you burn over a period of time. While we often think of exercising as burning calories, the effect of exercise is small compared to the total calories you burn – only about 20%.

When your heart beats, you breathe in and out, your body breaks down nutrients and makes new blood cells, you're burning calories. That's why you need an average of around 2,000 calories a day.

There are three basic biomolecules, also known as macronutrients, that your food can give you: proteins, carbohydrates, and fats. Food labels tell you exactly how much of each you're getting in a serving of food. The label also tells you how many grams of that food you need in a typical diet.

Depending on the label, the following are the major categories you'll find:

- Total calories per serving

- Grams of carbohydrates

- Grams of fat

- Milligrams of sodium

- Grams of protein

- Vitamins and minerals, if any

Within those major categories are some subdivisions to help you understand even more about what you're eating. Let's take a look at those subdivisions and what they mean for you when it comes to your diet.

Not All Carbohydrates Are Created Equal

When it comes to carbohydrates, some are better for you than others. Let's be clear – you need carbohydrates to have energy and to be healthy. Any diet that tells you to eliminate them completely is unhealthy.

A food label will break down carbohydrates into two categories – fiber and sugars. You need both. However, many people don't have enough fiber in their diets. You want to look for foods that are high in this nutrient.

Fiber helps you to lower your cholesterol and helps your digestive system to be more regular. You'll find more fiber in foods that contain whole grains such as wheat and oats. This is the healthier type of carbohydrate.

The other category of sugars is what you need to watch if you're concerned about diabetes. Depending on your situation with blood sugar, you'll want to limit how many grams of sugar you get in your diet.

When it comes to calories, every gram of carbohydrates contains 4 calories. So if you want to know how many calories in the food come from carbohydrates you can multiply your carbohydrate grams by four. Then you can look at the total calories in the serving to determine the percentage of calories that come from them.

The Purpose of Protein

Your body must have protein to build structures. Most of the structures inside you consist of protein and in order to have the building blocks to repair cells and develop muscles, you'll need to eat food that has this important molecule.

A food label will tell you the number of grams of protein in your food. You'll want to look for foods that are high in protein. Foods that have a lot of protein include nuts, meats, whole grain foods, and dairy products.

The Facts About Fats

Food labels will also give you information about fats. In the past, health practitioners told patients to avoid fat altogether. But it turns out that modern science doesn't support that type of diet. You actually need fats just like you need the other two macronutrients in your food.

The two major categories of fats are unsaturated and saturated. Unsaturated fats are the good ones that come from plant sources. At room temperature unsaturated fats stay liquid. These are considered healthy fats. You need them to help keep your skin and other organs healthy.

Unsaturated fats also help lower "bad" cholesterol and raise "good" cholesterol in your blood. This helps to protect your heart and prevent problems such as heart disease and stroke. They also help your digestive system to run smoothly.

Saturated fats come from animal fats. These are solid at room temperature and are considered unhealthy fats.

They contribute to high cholesterol, clogged arteries and can ultimately lead to heart disease, stroke, and other disorders.

Speaking of cholesterol, you can also find the amount of cholesterol in a serving of food on the label. Cholesterol amounts become important when you're trying to eat a heart healthy diet. If you're trying to lower cholesterol, you'll want to pay attention to this part of the label.

Trans fats are a category of fats that come from altering the chemical structure of an unsaturated fat. They are also called hydrogenated fats because the process of taking a liquid unsaturated fat to a solid trans fat involves adding hydrogen atoms to the molecules.

For many years it was thought that trans fats were as healthy as unsaturated fats, but that has been disproved. In fact, trans fats are actually more harmful than saturated fats. Because of the bad press, many food manufacturers are removing it from their products.

The United States Food and Drug Administration (FDA) now requires that trans fats are listed on food labels, if it is more than one gram per serving.

However if less than one gram, it does not have to be listed. The way to tell if a food has any trans fats in it or not is to take the grams of unsaturated and saturated fat, add them together and compare that number to the Total Fat listed. If they don't match, then the difference is trans fat not required to be listed.

It's a good idea to avoid any food that has trans fats in it. These fats have no nutritional value and are in fact harmful for you.

Sodium Safety

Another nutrient that food labels provide information about is sodium. Sodium is the fancy, scientific term for salt. If you have normal blood pressure, you probably don't pay too much attention to salt. But if you're suffering from high blood pressure, you can't ignore it.

Sodium causes your body to hold onto water and in turn raises your blood pressure. High blood pressure is a leading risk factor for heart disease and stroke. So if you have this issue, you need to check the labels. Speak with your doctor about what healthy amount of sodium is for you.

Then you'll want to look for labels that have low amounts of sodium or are even free from it. Some foods are labeled as "low sodium" but you still need to look at the label and see where it fits in with your needs.

Eating Vitamins and Minerals

While most people could use a multivitamin each day, the best way to get your vitamins and minerals is through the food you eat. In food, you find these vitamins and minerals in a natural state that's easy for your body to absorb.

Food labels will give you an idea of what nutrients can be found in a specific food. Look for foods that are high in vitamins and minerals such as calcium, vitamin C, vitamin A, potassium, and beta-carotene.

Making Time for Reading Food Labels

When you're new at reading food labels, it can seem overwhelming. But the more you do it, the easier it becomes. You'll also have your "go-to" foods that you can just pick up without revisiting the label every time.

Plan to spend some extra time at the grocery store when you're paying more attention to food labels. Pay attention to what nutrients you're looking to limit and what you need to add to your diet. Before you shop, make a list of what you need to get.

Then, as you're shopping, make a list of additional foods that you'd like to incorporate into your diet. You may also want to make a list of foods you'd like to avoid. Perhaps something you've always loved has way more cholesterol than you can afford. Spend some time looking for a substitute that's on the healthier side.

Understanding Ingredients

The other list you'll find on a nutrition label – or near it – is a list of ingredients. Ingredients on products are listed in order from greatest amount to least amount in the food. This list of ingredients can be very helpful for determining if a food is something you want to eat or not.

Some ingredients you might want to avoid include:

- Corn syrup (highly processed sugar)

- Hydrogenated oils

- Monosodium glutamate (MSG)

- Artificial coloring

- Artificial sweeteners (sucralose, aspartame, saccharin)

Ingredients that are not natural and come from chemical processing are generally not good for your body. A rule of thumb to follow is that if you can't pronounce the ingredient, you probably shouldn't eat it.

Once you start reading food labels, you'll be surprised to find out how many additives are in processed foods. While some foods with labels are healthy for you, there are a lot of foods that come in cans, boxes, and bags that contain harmful ingredients.

Foods Without Labels

When it comes to nutrition, the best thing you can do is look for foods that don't require labels. These are foods such as fruits, vegetables, and meats. The less processed your food is, the healthier it will be.

Other foods have labels, but are also close to their natural state. This includes food such as:

- Milk

- Yogurt

- Whole grain bread

- Whole grain cereals

- Natural peanut butter

- Natural cheese

When you're shopping, using food labels can help you to make good choices. Look for foods that are high in nutrition and low on saturated fats, artificial chemicals, cholesterol, and processed sugars. This will help you to prevent disease, have more energy, and even help you to shrink your waistline.

Sample Meals Cooking the TLC Way

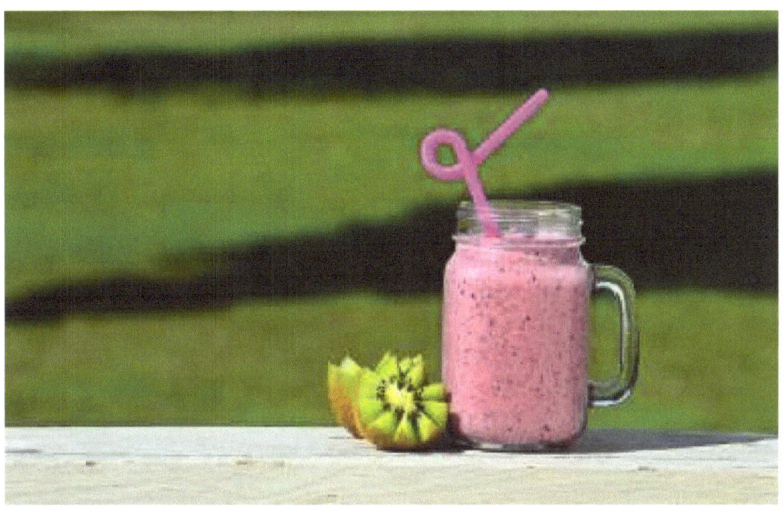

In this section, I'm going to introduce you to some delicious TLC recipes.

Breakfast Smoothie

Ingredients:

1 cup of fresh blueberries

½ cup of chopped baby spinach

1 cup of avocado, chopped

2 tbsp of almonds, minced 1 cup of coconut milk

½ cup of ice cubes (optional)

Preparation: Wash and drain the baby spinach. Combine with other ingredients in a blender and mix for about 30 seconds. Serve cold.

Fruit Salad

Ingredients:

1 cup of berries

½ cup of pineapple cubes

½ cup of chopped apple

5 mint springs

1 tbsp of fresh lime juice

1 tsp of lime zest ¼ cup of water

1 tsp of cinnamon

1 tsp of agave syrup

Preparation: In a small saucepan combine ¼ cup of water, mint spring, fresh lime juice and lime zest. Allow it to boil over medium temperature and cook for about 2-3 minutes. Remove from the heat and cool. Meanwhile, in a large bowl, combine 1 cup of berries, ½ cup of pineapple cubes and ½ cup of chopped apple. Add agave syrup and mix well. Pour the lime mixture over the salad and let it stand in the refrigerator for 20-30 minutes. Remove from the refrigerator and sprinkle with 1 tsp of cinnamon before serving.

Grilled Eggplant Slices With Chopped Fennel

Ingredients:

1 large eggplant

½ cup of chopped fennel

1 tbsp of olive oil

1 tsp of chopped parsley

Preparation: Peel the eggplant and cut into 3 equal slices. Bake it in a barbecue pan without oil. When done, spread olive oil over it, sprinkle with fennel and parsley. (These eggplant slices are great cold, so you can leave them overnight in a refrigerator)

Turkey Fillet With Walnuts And Maple Syrup

Ingredients:

3 turkey fillets

½ cup of walnuts

1 tsp of maple syrup

¼ cup of water

1 tbsp of olive oil salt to taste

Preparation: Fry the fillets in a barbecue pan, over a low temperature, for about 15 minutes, or until tender. Remove the pan from the heat and add water, maple syrup and walnuts.

Mix well and fry for another 5-6 minutes until the water evaporates. Stir constantly. Allow it to cool for a while before serving.

Beef Chop With Pineapple And Tumeric

Ingredients:

1.5 pounds of beef chop, boneless

2 tbsp of coconut oil

1 tbsp of olive oil

½ cup of coconut milk

1 tsp of tumeric

¼ tsp of pepper

1 medium pineapple, peeled and chopped

Preparation: Wash and dry the meat. Cut into bite size cubes. Combine the meat with coconut oil, coconut milk, tumeric, pepper and pineapple. Mix well and set side for 15 minutes. Use a large wok pan to heat up the olive oil. Remove te meat and pineapple chops from the marinade and fry for about 5-7 minutes on each side. Now pour in the remaining marinade, cover the wok pan and cook for 30 minutes over a medium temperature. The marinade will become thick and the meat soft. Remove from the heat and serve.

Salmon With Zucchini

Ingredients:

1 pound of sliced salmon fillets

2 small zucchinis

6 Brussels sprouts

3 tbsp of extra virgin olive oil

¼ tsp of pepper

Preparation: Peel and slice zucchinis into 0.5 inch thick circle shape slices. Cut salmon fillets into bite size pieces. Heat up one tbsp of olive oil in a large skillet and add your salmon fillets. Fry them up for about 10 minutes, or until they are nice and crispy. When done, move them to a plate covered with a kitchen paper to soak up the grease. Set aside.

Cut the Brussels sprouts in half. Combine with zucchini slices in a large bowl and add 2 tbsp of the remaining olive oil. Move the vegetables to the skillet and cook until the Brussel sprouts are tender. This should take no more than 10 minutes. Add your salmon fillets to the skillet, cover and allow it to rewarm. Serve and enjoy.

Making Smart Choice When Eating Away From Home

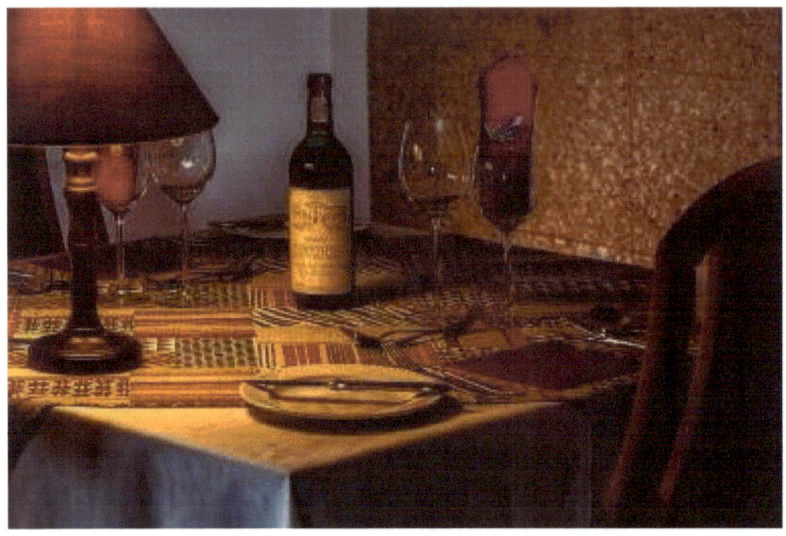

During the first couple of days of your TLC diet, you may be under the impression that it is difficult to follow. However, if you stick at it for longer than two weeks, it'll become easier and easier for you to follow, eventually becoming a habit after about 21 days.

As we mentioned earlier in the book, there may be times when you're too busy, or you may be going out with friends to a restaurant. During this time, you may be tempted to let the diet go.

The key to sticking with a healthy lifestyle diet is to prepare yourself for every possible situation you can think of. It is important that you try to make sure you always have access to healthy food, regardless. As long as you have healthy foods available at all times, you will be able to eat healthy.

This means you should take part in smart shopping, know how to cook your food and you should know exactly what to eat when you're eating out and attending social events.

Once you are able to handle all of that, it will be easy for you to eat healthily, regardless of where you may be. You're not going to have any excuses to run to the nearest fast food chain or eat chocolate (although dark chocolate is actually healthy to eat, but just one square at a time).

The way you cook is a big influence on how healthy your prepared food is going to be. The right cooking technique can make a health ingredient even healthier. On another note, the wrong technique can make things a lot worse. Take deep frying as an example – you're taking a vegetable and turning it into a giant sponge of fat. If you want to stay healthy, then you need to learn healthy cooking techniques.

Cooking Techniques

Cook using low-fat methods. Avoid using too much butter and oil. There are certain techniques that are preferred by advocates of the TLC diet.

These cooking techniques include:

- Grilling

- Steaming

- Boiling

- Roasting

- Baking

- Poaching

It is okay to sauté or even do some light frying, but keep your use of oil and butter low. You may want to invest in a good non-stick pan that will allow you to cook without using butter.

Eating Out On The TLC Diet

What you choose to eat during your outing all depends on the type of restaurant you choose.

Here, I am going to list Chinese restaurants and Italian as those seem to be pretty popular.

If you chose to eat out at a Chinese restaurant, stay away from the fried rice and go for food that doesn't contain MSG. Chinese cuisine consists of a lot of vegetables, but many times, their cooking styles are no good. Thankfully, on the menu, you'll be able to find barbecued, roasted and steamed food.

If you chose to eat out at an Italian restaurant, don't eat too much bread. When you choose bread as a side dish, it can be easy to overindulge. Eating too much, however, can do more harm than good. If you chose pizza, go for ones that are packed full of vegetable toppings and choose half the amount of cheese. Sometimes, these restaurants overload pizza with processed meat like pepperoni, bacon and sausage.

If you're going for pasta, choose the red sauce because this is healthier than any cream.

I'm going to tell you right now, if you want to be healthy, you need to get out there and get physical.

Regardless of your age, it's never too late for you to start exercising, so don't ever use your age as an excuse – there's 70 year old's out there doing extraordinary things with a bit of fitness!

In fact, the older you are, the more you should exercise. No, I'm not joking. Unless your doctor has advised against it, there's no reason not to. Exercise isn't going to have a negative impact on your body ... as a matter-of-fact, quite the opposite! Of course, before you get physically active, you should speak with your doctor to get the "go ahead," this way, you will feel better and have a better idea of your limitations.

You just need to learn how to fight through that laziness for the sake of your own health and get your body to start moving. Trust us, even the smallest of changes in your lifestyle can lead to a huge change in your body, so don't hesitate to start a good exercise regimen and stick to it.

At first, you're not going to like exercise, but eventually, as it becomes a part of your lifestyle, you're going to enjoy it.

Exercise – The Other TLC Diet Component

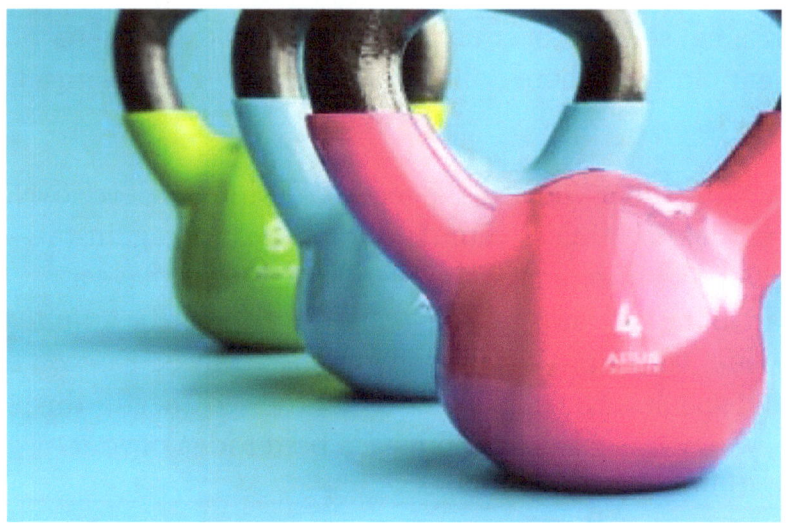

When coupled with healthy eating, exercising completes the TLC Diet. Losing weight is always a numbers game: burn 3,500 more calories per week than you eat and one pound of weight is gone. Unfortunately it only takes 2,200 more calories than you burn to gain a pound. Unfair I know, but that is the way it is. Exercising is your "ace-in-the-hole" when it comes to dieting and losing weight.

Types of Exercises

There are basically two types of exercises – cardio that works your cardiovascular system and strength training that works the muscles. Cardio training includes:

- Walking

- Jogging

- Swimming

- Biking

- Treadmill

- Elliptical trainer

- Rowing

Strength training includes:

- Weight lifting

- Using resistance bands

- Bodyweight (not using any additional weight)

As its name implies, it is for firming, toning and developing muscle mass and strength, depending on the type of moves, amount of weight or resistance and the number of repetitions and sets performed.

Yoga and Pilates are two other types of exercises, that are not really cardio or strength training pure, but more of a hybrid of the two. They tend to deal more physically with increasing joint movement, balance and flexibility, along with developing better breathing patterns. With meditation, they can even help the mind develop mentally and spiritually.

While these are the most popular, those are not the only types of exercise you can take part in. Honestly, you can easily create your own exercise routine that is fun for you. It can be pure one form or another, or it a hybrid of any of the three types.

Many people like to do cardio three days per week, strength training two days and Yoga or Pilates one day per week. Whatever program you set up, be sure to include at least one day of rest per week.

Just look on YouTube for at home exercise programs and you will find a multitude of fun and easy to perform programs.

Final Thoughts

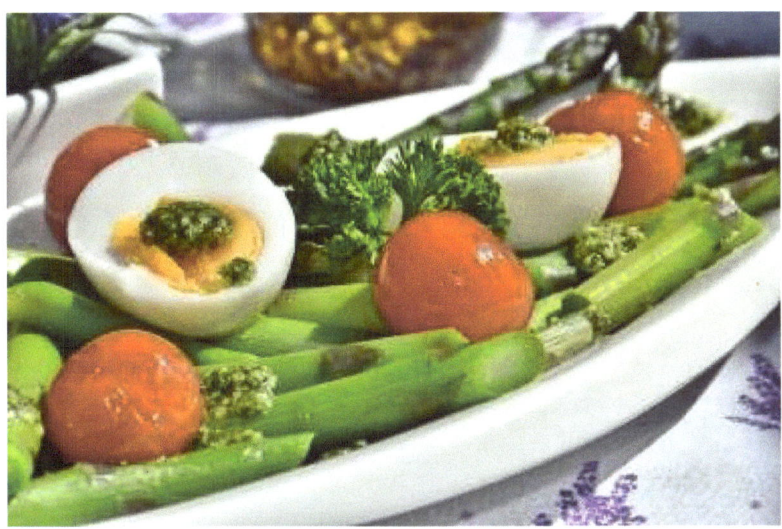

Well we have reached the pinnacle of our beginner's guide on the TLC Diet and I want to congratulate you for making it this far. In this final part we will summarize the main points we have covered so far and hopefully put to ease any questions or doubts you may have.

Tips To Start Today

At first, it's not going to be easy – no diet is easy, regardless of who you are, above all else however, the major thing to consider is sources of fat in your diet and monitoring saturated fat levels to lower your cholesterol.

While this seems difficult, after about a week or so, you'll start to pick up on the routine and before you know it, the TLC diet will naturally become a part of your lifestyle.

Here's a little bit of advice for you – put some time and effort into making your meals. You may even want to enroll in a nice yoga class (there may be one going on right now in your area). If you cannot find a yoga class, you can find many yoga videos online, which will allow you to practice yoga in the comfort of your own home.

Also, it may help if you have a nice support system going on. The more friends you have that will take part in this diet with you, the better off you're going to be.

In the end, don't let anything get in your way and remember the benefits of the TLC diet! You can also reward yourself. Rewarding yourself will give you something to look forward to. Just don't reward yourself with food – go for a new shirt or something along those lines.

Well that's it, you've reached the end. Wish you all the best in your journey to reduce your cholesterol levels by following the TLC diet.

Before moving on to reading the diet comparisons, consider what the father of medicine Hippocrates had to say:

"Let Food Be Thy Medicine And Medicine Be Thy Food"

How the TLC Diet Compares to Others

Losing weight and making changes to your life that have a good impact for your health is always a wise decision. There are many choices in diet plans that you can consider, depending on your specific health concerns.

You should always choose the kind of diet that focuses on foods that are good for you and one that has a goal of bringing things like blood pressure or bad cholesterol under control.

The TLC diet, which stands for **T**herapeutic **L**ifestyle **C**hanges, is one of the diets that can help you slim down as well as keep your blood pressure and cholesterol within a healthy number range.

It focuses on eating right, working out and keeping your weight at a number that's healthy for your height and age. It's rated one of the top 4 diets in the world and is especially strategic for those battling high cholesterol.

The TLC Diet versus the Biggest Loser Diet

The Biggest Loser Diet grew in popularity thanks to the show by the same name. But the quick weight loss does have drawbacks. People who tend to lose weight quickly don't always keep it off and this diet ranks lower in long term weight loss statistics than other diets do.

It's an extremely challenging diet, which makes it difficult for people to stick with. It's an expensive diet because of the foods that you'll buy. It mainly focuses on six weeks of hard exercising. In fact, some of the diet has people exercising for hours a day.

You'll be eating foods that you can buy from the grocery store and you don't have to buy any specialized meals just like with the TLC Diet. However, unlike the TLC Diet, you have to buy one of the books based on the Biggest Loser Diet so that you can follow the guidelines for the diet.

You'll be able to choose from more than one option in the books. Because of the hard emphasis placed on exercising, some people found that as soon as they stopped exercising, they did put back on the fast weight loss.

There's also a high potential for eating too little calories with this diet. It's always better to follow a life changing diet like given by the TLC Diet rather than a short term fix.

The TLC Diet versus the Engine 2 Diet

The name of this diet comes from the way it was established. It was a firefighter who came up with this diet and while it does have some good points, it is a heavily restricted diet as well as being ranked with a hard effort level.

It's a plant based diet, so you'll have to cut out animal products, dairy products and any foods that have a higher fat content than what the diet allows. The cost of the diet has a couple of options.

You can do it yourself and there is some help and guidance available for those who choose to use this diet. However, as far as any in depth support, that's only available if you pay for a membership.

So what you learn about the diet, you'll have to look up yourself or try to piece it together from others. The diet calls for you to get rid of every processed food you have in your kitchen.

While this isn't a bad idea, you'll also have to get rid of foods that contain over 2.5 grams of fat based on 100 calorie increments. So if you have a food product that's 100 calories but contains 3 grams of fat, you'll have to throw it away.

The good news is that the diet does work to help you lose weight as well as lower your cholesterol. The bad news is that you're not going to lose it in the healthiest way possible like with the TLC diet.

On the Engine 2 Diet, you may find yourself struggling to get the level of calcium that you need and you'll also have to take a vitamin B12 supplement since you won't be eating any meat products.

You might want to simply pursue the TLC diet and implement small changes, such as decreasing your dietary cholesterol to less than 200 mg a day for a 3-5% reduction in your bad cholesterol.

The TLC Diet versus Mediterranean Diet

One thing that you'll notice with the TLC diet is that it has a strong focus on the health of your body as a whole and rather than just weight loss alone. Instead of just giving you calorie levels to adhere to, you also have to maintain a level of exercise (30 minutes a day) to be successful.

If diabetes is an issue for you, then the TLC diet can help with that, too – since it helps more than any other diet to stabilize blood sugar levels. You'll benefit in many ways following this diet.

The Mediterranean Diet gets its name from the areas near the Mediterranean Sea. Like the TLC diet, the Mediterranean Diet encourages people to try to eat healthy. It suggests foods that are based on the eating style of those that live near the Sea.

On this diet, you would eat things like vegetables and fruits along with whole grains and lean meats. There's a strong focus on eating fish and using olive oil to give the foods their flavoring.

The Mediterranean Diet has some issues that can cause potential risks to your health. The first one is that there's such a strong focus on eating fish rather than consuming other meat.

While there is some truth to the health recommendation of not eating a lot of red meat, eating certain kinds of fish and seafood too often can give you too much mercury as well as other toxins.

Also, having wine daily is a staple of this diet and alcohol in any amount can cause damage to the cells in your liver as well as fatty liver disease if you overdo it.

The TLC diet has more of a plant sterol-based emphasis, making meat a rare inclusion of the meal plan. Your body will respond positively to the vegetables' ability to reduce high cholesterol numbers.

The TLC Diet versus DASH Diet

The DASH Diet stands for Dietary Approach to Stop Hypertension. Those who go on this diet will find themselves consuming meals that focus on eating things like fruits and vegetables, beans, poultry, whole grains, fish, nuts and dairy as long as it's low fat.

While you're on this diet, you'll need to learn about controlling your portions. You'll also have to learn about eating a wider array of foods than you might be used to.

The good news is that this diet is good for delivering the desired results if your goal is to lower your blood pressure. If you're someone who wants to jumpstart a weight loss plan, this one is not a fast start diet.

This diet takes a lot of time to not only learn about, but to put into effect as well because of the amount of food prep you'll face. If you're someone with a hectic schedule and don't have much extra time, this diet is probably not going to be the best choice for you.

With the TLC diet, you can either go all in at once, or make gradual changes that will deliver specific benefits toward lowering your cholesterol. For example, if you implement the recommendation of fiber additions to your diet, you'll see a 3-5% lowering of your cholesterol.

The TLC Diet versus Mayo Clinic Diet

When people hear the name Mayo Clinic, they immediately think a diet by the same name would have to be one that didn't have any downside to it. But the truth is that this diet is pretty simple.

What you get by following the diet is the same advice you get with most of the ones out there which is to eat less and exercise more. While that's pretty standard advice, it's not what most people are looking for.

They want to eat healthier but they want to know exactly how to do that in a way that will help them to lose weight and maintain that loss as well as provide other medical benefits, such as the lowering of bad cholesterol.

Unlike the TLC Diet, the Mayo Clinic Diet is not convenient. Unlike the TLC Diet, the meals are pretty detailed, many of them aren't quick to fix and they can involve expensive ingredients.

On top of that, some of the recipes associated with the diet aren't on par with medical advice pertaining to dieting. It's suggested that followers of the diet use egg substitute rather than eating real eggs.

The old, unproven claim is that real eggs are high in cholesterol and can cause heart disease. This advice is not only outdated and has been debunked but also has users consuming a processed food over real food by suggesting egg substitutes.

The diet pushes portion control but that's no different than most other diets. With the TLC diet, you can reduce your cholesterol 5-8% if you lose just 10 pounds of body weight.

This type of specific and measurable advice will help you hone in on the main health issues you have so that you can reap the benefits of making those changes.

The TLC Diet versus Vegetarian or Vegan Diet

There are many reasons that people choose the vegetarian or vegan diet. For some people, it has to do with wanting to be healthy. For others, it's about weight loss and for some, they just don't want to eat animal products.

Whatever your reason, there are some things that you should know about these diets versus the TLC diet before you commit to choosing your eating plan. The TLC diet can lower your cholesterol just like a vegetarian or vegan diet if that's your goal.

And it can do that while ensuring that the meals you eat are nutritionally sound as well as being tasty. But unlike the nutritional benefits from the food plan in the TLC diet, with the vegetarian or vegan diet, you miss out on important nutrients.

One of the problems with this type of diet is that most people don't get the protein load from plants that's found in animal products. The same kinds of vitamins and minerals found in meat can't be found in plants. One that's often lacking in vegetarian or vegan diets is Vitamin B12.

For people who choose to follow a vegan or vegetarian diet, it's recommended that they work with a dietician or other nutrition expert to make sure that their diet is healthy.

With the TLC diet, you can implement certain tips – such as adding 2 grams a day of plant sterols – to give you a 5-15% LDL reduction. It's more about what to add in some cases than it is about what to give up.

The TLC Diet versus Flexitarian Diet

There's a diet that people enjoy following when they want to have a vegetarian diet that's based on plants as the main staple food source, but also want to be able to eat meat if they want to have it. This diet is called the Flexitarian Diet.

While it looks pretty good on the surface when you think about eating fruits and vegetables along with the nuts and legumes, you have to take a deeper look to see just what this diet is all about.

It calls for heavy calorie restrictions that, according to health guidelines, don't offer enough calorie consumption to be considered good for you. In fact, the low calorie count can lead to episodes of low blood sugar.

Unlike the TLC diet, this one doesn't make sure that you get the proper amount of food that you need. To follow the eating plan, you have to buy a guide book to lead you through the steps of how to eat on this diet.

While it might be a diet for people who want some meat but not a lot, as a whole, this diet doesn't stack up well against the TLC diet. You can implement a portion of the TLC diet that tells you to decrease saturated fat to less than 7% of your calories and you'll enjoy an 8-10% reduction in your LDL levels!

The TLC Diet versus Weight Watchers

Weight Watchers has been around for many years and boasts of many success stories. The diet focus is on nutritionally sound foods, yet no foods, including those that aren't all that healthy, are off limits.

There is a focus on eating foods based on certain points and counting how the food ranks. This is a definite negative for the program because the focus is on labeling food using a points system.

Users can count up their points to see how much they have left to eat for the day. This doesn't effectively teach anything about nutritional values. There may be a lack of nutritional needs being met by those who follow Weight Watchers.

Some people buy the frozen meals offered by Weight Watchers and just eat those thinking that this way is healthy, but fresh food sources are always more nutritionally sound than frozen ones.

The TLC Diet versus the Dean Ornish Diet

There are a few ways that you can use this diet to lose weight and get healthier. You can completely change your eating lifestyle from top to bottom or you can make some small changes that can make a difference in how you look and feel.

While it's not too much of a challenging diet, it's not as easy as others that are available either. The concept of this diet is that it can be used to shed excess pounds but also to reverse certain health conditions such as diabetes or high cholesterol.

It's considered a preventative diet for some diseases as well. To go on this diet, you would follow the guidelines given for the different groups of food which are ranked according to group 1 to group 5.

The problem with the diet is that it strictly limits proteins and encourages followers to limit meats - even lean, unprocessed meats that should be a part of a healthy diet as encouraged by the TLC Diet.

There is a focus on plant based foods, which can often cause a nutritional lack of certain vitamins and minerals. The foods suggested are vegetables, fruits, grains and beans while limiting dairy products.

Following certain guidelines suggested in the diet such as eating organic foods can be too expensive for some dieters.

The best thing you can do if you're suffering from high cholesterol is implement the various steps within the TLC Diet and test your cholesterol after each one to see how big the changes were. Keep going until your health issues have been resolved and new habits have replaced the old ones!

Other Relevant Books by This Author

If you would like to read more relevant books about this topic, here is a list of the CreateSpace links, titles and descriptions from this author:

https://www.createspace.com/6594833

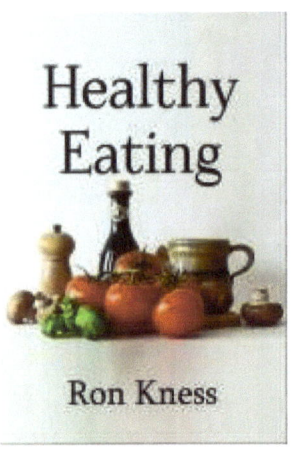

Healthy Eating: Making Smart Food Choices for Health and Longevity

We all want to be healthy. Good health, like most things worth having, requires some effort. That effort best begins with self-education. Living a healthy lifestyle starts with what you eat. After all, "we are what we eat"!

We are made personally aware of this statement when we over-indulge in poor food and drink choices. As our body deals with the consequences we feel sluggish, nauseous, irritable and lacking in energy and enthusiasm.

In modern western societies, we live in a world where our food health is usually compromised more by excess quantity than scarcity. It seems like almost all of the fast food chains have their own form of "supersizing". However, it is critical to make a distinction between sufficient or even excess food consumption and adequate nutrient intake.

In other words, more food doesn't necessarily mean it is better for you nutritionally. In fact, much of the food and drink we consume are nothing more than empty calories – calories containing very few, if any, nutrients.

The bottom line is most foods are produced with continuing and increasing sales as the major driver. How good they are for you isn't even part of the equation. To achieve this, producers and manufacturers often place more emphasis on taste, texture and appearance and shelf life rather than nutrient availability.

Good food can and does taste good, but clever processing can make foods with little nutrient value taste incredibly good too. It is up to you to know the difference and that is where this information will help you to understand why some foods and food types are better for your health, vitality and well-being. Let's get started.

https://www.createspace.com/6845571

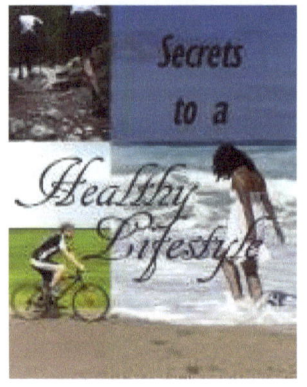

Secrets to a Healthy Lifestyle: 7 Lifestyle Changes To Make This Year the Best Yet

Along with a New Year comes the opportunity to let go of the past and start fresh and anew. It's a perfect time to get serious about getting healthy. Don't think of it as a new year's resolution. Think of it as a brand-new start on your life.

Out with the old, and in with the new. What's more is that it's not as difficult as you think. You can have less stress with a few simple daily actions, eat better by adding in more healthy food and get healthier by exercising more without feeling like it's so much work.

In addition, just a few money and time management, and unhealthy habit changes will make all the difference in your life. Finally, you'll have more time for more fun without spending tons of money.

You're going to feel so much better with just a few specific changes, that you'll have the very best year you've ever had.

Turn off electronics, head for a walk in the park, have a picnic, then go grocery shopping leisurely. Make fun a priority in your life and you'll naturally be healthier, happier and have an amazing year, every year.

https://www.createspace.com/6923372

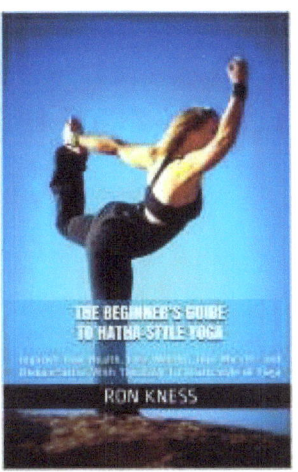

The Beginner's Guide to Hatha-Style Yoga: Improve Your Health, Lose Weight, Tone Muscles and Reduce Stress With This Easy-To-Learn Style of Yoga

We want there to be a calmness of in both our mind and spirit. We also want to be healthier as we age. And to accomplish both, we must learn to do the poses of Hatha yoga!

We can achieve ALL of these goals with the newest release from Ron Kness called "The Beginner's Guide To Hatha-Style Yoga".

Based on these exciting teachings, you will learn about all the dramatic benefits of doing Hatha yoga like improved health, weight loss, muscle toning and reducing stress, along with improved flexibility and balance.

This book is built around a very clear, concept: learn yoga and reap the benefits from doing this style of yoga - Hatha.

It's not just about learning how to do this easy-to-learn style of yoga. Having great overall health is linked to being in charge and making smart healthy lifestyle decisions. This is because learning how to do any style of yoga should be part of any healthy lifestyle.

In this book, we look at all of the ways you can improve your own overall health, starting with deciding to learn the poses and practice yoga. This book will also look at the many other steps that can be taken to support this goal, like viewing the suggested videos of poses used in Hatha yoga depending on the health benefit you want to gain.

The choices you make about joining a Hatha yoga class or learning it by yourself and doing it at home has a great impact on your overall health.

In "The Beginner's Guide To Hatha-Style Yoga", we'll cover all the bases, giving you everything you need to know to do this style of yoga that provides the health benefits mentioned.

Get your copy now and start improving your health tomorrow!

About the Author

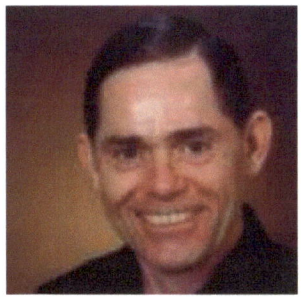

I have published over 125 books on Amazon for Kindle, CreateSpace and other publishing platforms.

While most of my books are on health and fitness in general, as I age (now 65) at the time of this writing) my topics of interest are geared toward aging baby boomers and older.

Besides my own writing, I also ghostwrite ebooks, books, reports, articles, blogs and do Kindle conversions for clients on a variety of topics.

Today my wife and I are retired from our careers and live in Gold Canyon, AZ. I now write as a retirement business where you'll find me happily sitting in my office typing away on my laptop as I work on my next book or ghostwriting project . . . that is if we are not traveling on a cruise ship - our new-found mode of travel.